STAYING HEALTHY

IN

PREGNANCY

DR. Tracy E. Gagnon

I. Introduction

- Explanation of pregnancy and the changes that occur in the body
- Importance of staying healthy during pregnancy
- Overview of the three trimesters

II. First Trimester

- Explanation of the changes that occur during the first trimester
- Hormonal changes and their effects on the body
- Common symptoms and how to manage them
- Nutritional needs and dietary recommendations
- Exercise and physical activity recommendations

III. Second Trimester

- Explanation of the changes that occur during the second trimester
- Hormonal changes and their effects on the body
- Common symptoms and how to manage them
- Nutritional needs and dietary recommendations
- Exercise and physical activity recommendations

IV. Third Trimester

- Explanation of the changes that occur during the third trimester
- Hormonal changes and their effects on the body
- Common symptoms and how to manage them

- Nutritional needs and dietary recommendations
- Exercise and physical activity recommendations

V. Hormonal Imbalance during Pregnancy

- Explanation of hormonal changes during pregnancy and their effects on the body
- Common hormonal imbalances during pregnancy and their symptoms
- How to manage hormonal imbalances during pregnancy

VI. Complications during Pregnancy

- Overview of common complications during pregnancy
- Signs and symptoms of complications
- Treatment options for complications
- Prevention strategies for complications

VII. Tips for Staying Healthy During Pregnancy

- Importance of regular prenatal care
- Maintaining a healthy diet and exercise routine
- Managing stress and getting enough rest
- Avoiding harmful substances and environmental factors

VIII. Conclusion

- Summary of key points
- Importance of staying healthy during pregnancy for the mother and baby

- Encouragement to seek medical advice and support during pregnancy

Introduction

Pregnancy is a special time in a woman's life when she experiences various physical and emotional changes. It is important to stay healthy during this time to ensure the well-being of both the mother and the baby. Pregnancy is divided into three trimesters, each with its unique set of changes and challenges. Hormonal imbalance is also a common experience during pregnancy that can affect a woman's physical and emotional well-being. This guide will provide an overview of pregnancy and how to stay healthy during each trimester, as well as how to manage hormonal imbalances and prevent complications. Additionally, it will provide tips for maintaining a healthy lifestyle during pregnancy and the importance of seeking medical advice and support.

Explanation of pregnancy and the changes that occur in the body

Pregnancy is a process where a woman's body undergoes significant changes to support the growth and development of a fetus. These changes are mainly due to hormonal fluctuations, which are necessary to support the pregnancy. Some of the changes that occur during pregnancy include:

1. Growth of the Uterus: The uterus grows rapidly during pregnancy to accommodate the growing fetus. This growth can cause discomfort, including abdominal cramps and backaches.
2. Weight Gain: Pregnant women usually gain weight as the baby grows. This weight gain is essential for a healthy pregnancy but can cause physical discomfort and affect self-esteem.
3. Breast Changes: Breast changes are common during pregnancy. The breasts become larger and more sensitive due to hormonal changes, which prepare them for breastfeeding.
4. Digestive Changes: Hormonal changes during pregnancy can slow down digestion, leading to constipation, heartburn, and other digestive issues.
5. Skin Changes: Hormonal changes can cause skin changes during pregnancy, including acne, stretch marks, and darkening of the skin around the nipples, face, and abdomen.
6. Emotional Changes: Pregnancy can also cause emotional changes due to hormonal fluctuations. Pregnant women may experience mood swings, anxiety, and depression.

It is important to understand these changes and how they can affect a woman's physical and emotional well-being during pregnancy. With proper care and attention, many of these changes can be managed effectively.

Importance of staying healthy during pregnancy

Staying healthy during pregnancy is essential for both the mother and the baby's well-being. A healthy pregnancy reduces the risk of complications and promotes healthy fetal development. Some of the benefits of staying healthy during pregnancy include:

1. Reduced Risk of Complications: A healthy pregnancy reduces the risk of complications such as preterm labor, gestational diabetes, high blood pressure, and preeclampsia. These complications can be dangerous for both the mother and the baby.
2. Healthy Fetal Development: A healthy pregnancy provides the best possible environment for fetal growth and development. Proper nutrition, exercise, and prenatal care are crucial for ensuring the baby's healthy development.
3. Improved Maternal Health: Staying healthy during pregnancy can improve a woman's overall health and well-being. It can reduce the risk of postpartum depression and promote a faster recovery after delivery.
4. Better Birth Outcomes: A healthy pregnancy can lead to better birth outcomes, including a lower risk of preterm birth, low birth weight, and stillbirth.

To stay healthy during pregnancy, it is important to maintain a healthy lifestyle, including proper nutrition, regular exercise, and regular prenatal care. It is also essential to avoid harmful substances such as tobacco, alcohol, and drugs, which can negatively impact fetal development and lead to complications during pregnancy.

Overview of the three trimesters

Pregnancy is typically divided into three trimesters, each lasting about three months. Each trimester is characterized by different physical and emotional changes for the mother and the growing fetus.

First Trimester (Weeks 1-12) The first trimester is a crucial time for fetal development, as the baby's major organs and systems begin to form. During this time, the mother may experience symptoms such as morning sickness, fatigue, and breast tenderness. Hormonal changes can also cause mood swings and changes in appetite. Prenatal care is essential during the first trimester to monitor fetal development, screen for any potential complications, and provide support to the mother.

Second Trimester (Weeks 13-28) The second trimester is often considered the "honeymoon period" of pregnancy. The mother's energy levels may improve, and she may experience less nausea and fatigue. The fetus continues to grow and develop, and the mother may begin to feel fetal movements. Prenatal care during the second trimester includes regular check-ups, ultrasounds to monitor fetal growth, and screening tests for genetic disorders.

Third Trimester (Weeks 29-40+) During the third trimester, the fetus continues to grow and develop, and the mother may experience discomfort as the baby puts pressure on her organs and muscles. The mother may experience symptoms such as back pain, frequent urination, and difficulty sleeping. The baby may move into the head-down position in preparation for delivery. Prenatal care during the third trimester includes monitoring fetal growth, testing for Group B streptococcus, and discussing birth options with the healthcare provider.

Overall, each trimester is a unique experience for both the mother and the growing fetus. Proper prenatal care and a healthy lifestyle are essential for promoting healthy fetal development and ensuring a safe and healthy delivery.

First Trimester

The first trimester of pregnancy is a crucial time for fetal development, as the baby's major organs and systems begin to form. The first trimester lasts from week 1 to week 12 of pregnancy. During this time, the mother may experience a range of physical and emotional changes as her body adapts to the pregnancy.

One of the most common symptoms experienced during the first trimester is morning sickness, which can involve nausea and vomiting. This is caused by hormonal changes in the body and can be managed through dietary changes, such as eating smaller, more frequent meals, and avoiding foods that trigger nausea.

Fatigue is also a common symptom during the first trimester, as the body is working hard to support the developing fetus. Getting plenty of rest and practicing good sleep hygiene can help manage fatigue.

The mother's breasts may become tender and sore during the first trimester as they prepare for breastfeeding. Hormonal changes can also cause mood swings and changes in appetite. It is important for the mother to eat a healthy, balanced diet and take prenatal vitamins to support the developing fetus.

Prenatal care is essential during the first trimester to monitor fetal development, screen for any potential complications, and provide support to the mother. The healthcare provider will typically schedule an initial prenatal visit around 8 weeks of pregnancy to confirm the pregnancy and assess the mother's health.

The healthcare provider will also screen for any risk factors or medical conditions that could impact the pregnancy, such as high blood pressure or gestational diabetes. Additional prenatal testing may be recommended based on the mother's age, medical history, or family history.

Overall, the first trimester is a critical time for fetal development, and proper prenatal care is essential for promoting a healthy pregnancy and a safe delivery. It is important for the mother to take care of her own physical and emotional needs during this time, and to seek support from her healthcare provider and loved ones as needed.

Explanation of the changes that occur during the first trimester

During the first trimester of pregnancy, the body undergoes many changes as it adapts to support the developing fetus. These changes are caused by hormonal shifts and the physical demands of pregnancy.

One of the earliest signs of pregnancy is a missed menstrual period, which occurs when the fertilized egg implants in the uterus. This triggers a surge in hormones, including human chorionic gonadotropin (hCG), which can cause pregnancy symptoms such as fatigue, breast tenderness, and nausea.

The uterus begins to enlarge during the first trimester to accommodate the growing fetus. As a result, the mother may experience mild cramping and a feeling of fullness or heaviness in the pelvic area.

The placenta, which provides nutrients and oxygen to the fetus, also begins to form during the first trimester. This structure attaches to the uterine wall and contains blood vessels that allow for the exchange of gases and nutrients between the mother and fetus.

The baby's major organs and systems begin to form during the first trimester. By the end of the first trimester, the fetus has a beating heart, and its brain, nervous system, digestive system, and other organs have started to develop.

However, the first trimester is also a time of increased risk for miscarriage, particularly in the first few weeks of pregnancy. It is important for the mother to take care of her physical and emotional health, avoid harmful substances such as alcohol and tobacco, and seek prompt medical care if she experiences any symptoms of complications such as bleeding or cramping.

Overall, the changes that occur during the first trimester are essential for the development of a healthy fetus, but they can also be challenging for the mother. It is important for the mother to take care of her own needs and seek support from her healthcare provider and loved ones as needed.

Hormonal changes and their effects on the body

During the first trimester of pregnancy, there are significant hormonal changes that occur in the body to support the growth and development of the fetus. These hormonal changes can have various effects on the mother's body and can cause pregnancy symptoms.

One of the main hormones that increases during the first trimester is human chorionic gonadotropin (hCG), which is produced by the placenta. HCG is responsible for maintaining the pregnancy and can cause nausea and vomiting, commonly known as morning sickness, in the mother.

Progesterone is another hormone that increases during the first trimester. This hormone helps to thicken and prepare the uterus for implantation and provides support to the growing fetus. However, progesterone can also cause side effects such as fatigue, constipation, and bloating.

Estrogen levels also increase during the first trimester. This hormone helps to stimulate the growth of the uterus and prepares the breasts for milk production. However, estrogen can also cause breast tenderness, mood swings, and headaches in some women.

During the first trimester, the body also produces higher levels of relaxin, a hormone that helps to relax the muscles and ligaments in the pelvis to prepare for childbirth. This can cause joint pain and discomfort in the hips and lower back for some women.

Overall, hormonal changes during the first trimester are a necessary part of supporting the developing fetus, but they can also cause discomfort and pregnancy symptoms for the mother. It is important for the mother to take care of her physical and emotional health during this time and seek support from her healthcare provider as needed.

Common symptoms and how to manage them

Some common symptoms during the first trimester of pregnancy include:

1. Nausea and vomiting: This is commonly referred to as morning sickness and is caused by the increased levels of hCG in the body. To manage this symptom, it is recommended to eat small, frequent meals throughout the day, avoid foods and smells that trigger nausea, and stay hydrated.
2. Fatigue: Increased levels of progesterone can cause fatigue during the first trimester. To manage this symptom, it is recommended to get plenty of rest and sleep, and to stay physically active through moderate exercise.
3. Breast tenderness: Increased levels of estrogen can cause breast tenderness during the first trimester. To manage this symptom, it is recommended to wear a supportive bra, avoid caffeine and alcohol, and use warm compresses to alleviate discomfort.
4. Constipation: Increased levels of progesterone can cause constipation during the first trimester. To manage this symptom, it is recommended to eat a high-fiber diet, stay hydrated, and engage in regular physical activity.
5. Mood swings: Hormonal changes during the first trimester can cause mood swings in some women. To manage this symptom, it is recommended to practice relaxation techniques such as meditation or yoga, seek support from friends and family, and talk to a healthcare provider if needed.

It is important to note that while some discomfort is normal during the first trimester, certain symptoms such as severe nausea and vomiting or vaginal bleeding should be reported to a healthcare provider immediately.

Overall, taking care of physical and emotional health is essential during the first trimester of pregnancy to support the health and development of the growing fetus.

Nutritional needs and dietary recommendations

During the first trimester, it is important to ensure proper nutrition to support the healthy development of the fetus. Here are some dietary recommendations for pregnant women:

1. Folic acid: Folic acid is a B vitamin that is essential for the healthy development of the neural tube in the fetus. It is recommended to take a prenatal vitamin containing at least 400 mcg of folic acid daily.
2. Iron: Iron is essential for the formation of red blood cells, which carry oxygen to the fetus. It is recommended to consume iron-rich foods such as lean red meat, poultry, fish, beans, and fortified cereals.
3. Calcium: Calcium is important for the development of strong bones and teeth in the fetus. It is recommended to consume calcium-rich foods such as dairy products, fortified juices, and leafy greens.
4. Protein: Protein is essential for the growth and development of the fetus. It is recommended to consume protein-rich foods such as lean meats, fish, poultry, beans, and nuts.
5. Healthy fats: Healthy fats such as omega-3 fatty acids are important for the development of the fetal brain and nervous system. It is recommended to consume fatty fish such as salmon, nuts, and seeds.

In addition to these dietary recommendations, it is important to stay hydrated and avoid alcohol, caffeine, and raw or undercooked meats and fish. It is also recommended to consult with a healthcare provider for personalized nutrition recommendations during pregnancy.

Overall, maintaining a balanced and nutritious diet during the first trimester can support the health and development of the growing fetus.

Exercise and physical activity recommendations

During the first trimester, it is generally safe for women to continue their regular exercise routine if they feel up to it. However, it is important to avoid high-impact activities and movements that could result in falls or injury to the abdomen. Low-impact exercises such as walking, swimming, and prenatal yoga are good options for staying active during pregnancy.

It is important to listen to your body during this time and not push yourself too hard. If you feel fatigued or experience nausea, it is okay to take a break from exercise and rest. It is also important to stay hydrated and to avoid becoming overheated during exercise.

Women should consult with their healthcare provider before beginning any exercise program during pregnancy to ensure that it is safe for them and their baby. In some cases, women with high-risk pregnancies or certain medical conditions may be advised to avoid exercise or to modify their routine.

Overall, staying active during pregnancy can have many benefits, including improved mood, better sleep, and increased energy levels. Exercise can also help to prepare the body for labor and delivery.

Second Trimester

The second trimester is often referred to as the "golden trimester" as many women experience relief from the symptoms that were common during the first trimester. However, there are still important considerations for staying healthy during this time.

Here are some key points to keep in mind:

- Changes in the body: During the second trimester, the uterus continues to expand and the baby grows rapidly. This can result in back pain, pelvic pressure, and other physical discomforts. Some women may also experience stretch marks or varicose veins.
- Hormonal changes: Hormonal changes during the second trimester can result in increased blood volume, which can cause swelling in the feet and ankles.
- Nutritional needs: It is important to continue eating a healthy, balanced diet during the second trimester. Women should aim to consume a variety of nutrient-dense foods and stay hydrated.

- Exercise: As long as there are no medical complications, women can continue to exercise during the second trimester. However, some modifications may be necessary as the belly grows. Prenatal yoga, swimming, and walking are all good options.
- Preparing for childbirth: During the second trimester, women may want to start thinking about childbirth education classes and creating a birth plan.
- Mental health: Pregnancy can be an emotional time, and women may experience a range of feelings during the second trimester. It is important to prioritize mental health and seek support if needed.

Overall, the second trimester is a time for continued self-care and preparation for childbirth.

Explanation of the changes that occur during the second trimester

During the second trimester, which lasts from week 13 to week 28, the developing fetus grows rapidly, and the mother's body undergoes significant changes. Some of the notable changes during this stage include:

1. Fetal development: During the second trimester, the fetus grows from about the size of a lemon to around 14 inches in length and 2 pounds in weight. The fetus begins to develop organs, including the liver, kidneys, and lungs, and bones start to harden.
2. Maternal body changes: The uterus expands to accommodate the growing fetus, which may cause back

pain, constipation, and urinary frequency. The mother may also experience increased appetite, weight gain, and changes in skin pigmentation.
3.   Hormonal changes: Hormonal changes continue during the second trimester, but the levels of hormones such as estrogen and progesterone stabilize.
4.   Emotional changes: Many women report feeling more energetic and less nauseous during the second trimester, which may lead to an improved emotional state.
5.   Increased fetal movement: The mother may start to feel the fetus moving regularly during this stage.
6.   Health assessments: During the second trimester, the mother may have a range of health assessments, including ultrasound scans and glucose screening for gestational diabetes.

It's important to continue to prioritize healthy habits during the second trimester to support fetal growth and development and maintain maternal health.

Hormonal changes and their effects on the body

During the second trimester, hormonal changes continue to occur in the pregnant person's body. The placenta begins to produce hormones, including estrogen and progesterone, which help maintain the pregnancy and prepare the body for childbirth.

Estrogen levels increase during the second trimester, which can cause the following changes:

1. Skin changes: Some pregnant people experience an increase in skin pigmentation, such as darkening of the skin around the nipples, on the face, or on the linea nigra (a dark line that runs from the navel to the pubic bone).
2. Hair changes: Some pregnant people experience thicker, fuller hair during the second trimester due to increased levels of estrogen.
3. Joint laxity: The hormone relaxin, which is produced during pregnancy, causes the ligaments and joints to become more relaxed, which can increase the risk of injury.

Progesterone levels also continue to rise during the second trimester. This hormone helps relax the muscles in the uterus, which can reduce the risk of premature labor.

Overall, the hormonal changes during the second trimester are important for supporting the growth and development of the fetus, as well as preparing the pregnant person's body for childbirth.

Common symptoms and how to manage them

During the second trimester, many of the symptoms from the first trimester may subside or become less severe. However, new symptoms may arise as the baby continues to grow and develop. Some common symptoms during the second trimester include:

1. Back pain: As the baby grows, the mother's center of gravity shifts forward, which can put extra strain on the lower back. Practicing good posture and doing exercises to strengthen the back muscles can help alleviate back pain.
2. Leg cramps: Leg cramps can be caused by the extra weight and pressure on the legs, as well as changes in circulation. Gentle stretching exercises, staying hydrated, and avoiding standing for long periods of time can help reduce the frequency and severity of leg cramps.
3. Heartburn and indigestion: Hormonal changes during pregnancy can cause the muscles in the digestive tract to relax, which can lead to heartburn and indigestion. Eating small, frequent meals and avoiding spicy, fatty, or fried foods can help alleviate these symptoms.
4. Swelling: As the body retains more water during pregnancy, swelling can occur in the feet, ankles, and hands. Elevating the legs and wearing comfortable, supportive shoes can help reduce swelling.
5. Skin changes: Hormonal changes can cause changes in the skin, such as darkening of the areolas, a linea nigra (a dark line that can appear on the belly), and the appearance of stretch marks. Using moisturizer and avoiding exposure to the sun can help minimize these changes.
6. Increased appetite and weight gain: As the baby grows, the mother's appetite may increase, leading to weight gain. It's important to continue eating a healthy, balanced diet and to exercise regularly to help manage weight gain and promote overall health.
7. Braxton Hicks contractions: These are practice contractions that can occur during the second trimester and become more frequent as the pregnancy progresses. They are usually painless and can help prepare the body for labor.

Managing these symptoms may involve similar strategies to those used during the first trimester, such as maintaining a healthy diet and exercise routine, staying hydrated, and getting plenty of rest. It's also important to attend regular prenatal checkups to monitor the baby's growth and development.

Nutritional needs and dietary recommendations

During the second trimester, the baby's growth accelerates, and it becomes important to maintain a healthy diet to support their development. The recommended weight gain during this trimester is around 1 pound per week. Here are some nutritional needs and dietary recommendations during the second trimester:

1. Protein: Protein is essential for the growth and development of the baby's organs and tissues. Pregnant women should aim to consume around 75-100 grams of protein per day. Good sources of protein include meat, poultry, fish, beans, lentils, tofu, and dairy products.
2. Iron: Iron is important for the formation of red blood cells, which carry oxygen to the baby. During the second trimester, the recommended daily intake of iron is 27 milligrams. Good sources of iron include lean red meat, poultry, fish, beans, lentils, tofu, and fortified breakfast cereals.
3. Calcium: Calcium is important for the development of the baby's bones and teeth. Pregnant women should aim to consume around 1,000 milligrams of calcium per day. Good

sources of calcium include dairy products, leafy greens, fortified cereals, and calcium-fortified orange juice.

4. Fruits and vegetables: Fruits and vegetables are a good source of vitamins, minerals, and fiber. Pregnant women should aim to consume at least 2 cups of fruits and 2.5 cups of vegetables per day. Colorful fruits and vegetables are particularly good sources of antioxidants, which can help protect against cell damage.

5. Water: Staying hydrated is important during pregnancy, as it helps prevent constipation, flushes out toxins, and supports the baby's development. Pregnant women should aim to drink at least 8-10 glasses of water per day.

6. Avoid certain foods: Pregnant women should avoid certain foods that may be harmful to the baby, including raw or undercooked meat, fish high in mercury, unpasteurized dairy products, and certain types of seafood.

It's important to talk to a healthcare provider or a registered dietitian for personalized recommendations on nutrition during pregnancy.

Exercise and physical activity recommendations

During the second trimester, most women feel more energetic and less nauseated than in the first trimester. This is a good time to focus on staying active and healthy to support the growth and development of the fetus. Here are some exercise and physical activity recommendations for the second trimester:

1. Low-impact exercises: As your belly grows, high-impact exercises can become uncomfortable and potentially harmful. Opt for low-impact exercises such as walking, swimming, prenatal yoga, and cycling on a stationary bike.
2. Strengthening exercises: Focus on exercises that strengthen your muscles, such as squats, lunges, and bicep curls using light weights or resistance bands. Strengthening your muscles can help prepare your body for the physical demands of childbirth.
3. Pelvic floor exercises: These exercises can help prevent urinary incontinence and prepare your pelvic muscles for childbirth. To perform pelvic floor exercises, squeeze the muscles around your vagina and anus as if you are trying to stop the flow of urine. Hold for a few seconds and release.
4. Avoid overheating: During pregnancy, your body temperature is already slightly elevated, so avoid exercising in hot and humid environments. Make sure to drink plenty of water before, during, and after exercise.
5. Listen to your body: If you feel tired or experience any discomfort, it's okay to take a break or modify your exercise routine. Always listen to your body and consult your healthcare provider if you have any concerns.

Third Trimester

The third trimester is the final stage of pregnancy, which typically lasts from week 28 until delivery, which can occur anytime between weeks 37 and 42. During this time, the baby continues to grow and develop rapidly, and the mother's body prepares for labor and delivery.

Some of the changes that occur during the third trimester include:

1. Fetal growth and development: The baby's brain and nervous system continue to develop rapidly, and their lungs and other organs become more mature.
2. Weight gain: The mother may continue to gain weight, with most of the weight gain occurring in the third trimester as the baby grows.
3. Braxton Hicks contractions: These are practice contractions that can occur in the third trimester, which help to prepare the body for labor.
4. Increased fatigue: As the body works harder to support the growing baby, the mother may feel more tired and fatigued.
5. Swelling: The feet, ankles, and hands may become swollen due to increased fluid retention.

Hormonal changes during the third trimester include a further increase in the levels of progesterone and estrogen, which help to prepare the body for labor and delivery.

Common symptoms during the third trimester include:

1. Braxton Hicks contractions
2. Back pain
3. Increased fatigue
4. Shortness of breath
5. Heartburn
6. Swelling

Nutritional needs during the third trimester include an increase in the intake of protein, calcium, and iron. It is also important to stay hydrated by drinking plenty of water.

Exercise during the third trimester should focus on low-impact activities such as walking, swimming, or prenatal yoga. It is important to listen to your body and avoid any exercises that cause discomfort or pain.

During the third trimester, it is important to prepare for labor and delivery by attending childbirth classes, discussing birth preferences with your healthcare provider, and packing a hospital bag. It is also important to monitor fetal movements and report any changes or concerns to your healthcare provider.

Explanation of the changes that occur during the third trimester

During the third trimester, which begins at 28 weeks and ends at birth, the fetus continues to grow rapidly, and the mother's body prepares for labor and delivery. Some of the changes that occur during the third trimester include:

1. Fetal growth: The fetus gains weight rapidly during the third trimester, and it may move less often due to the limited space in the uterus.
2. Braxton Hicks contractions: These are practice contractions that help the uterus prepare for labor. They can be uncomfortable, but they are usually not painful.

3. Shortness of breath: As the uterus expands and presses against the diaphragm, it can become difficult to breathe deeply.
4. Frequent urination: The growing uterus puts pressure on the bladder, causing the need to urinate more often.
5. Swelling: Many women experience swelling in the feet, ankles, and hands during the third trimester.
6. Fatigue: As the body prepares for labor and delivery, many women experience increased fatigue and may have trouble sleeping.
7. Braxton Hicks contractions: These are practice contractions that help the uterus prepare for labor. They can be uncomfortable, but they are usually not painful.
8. Backache: As the baby grows and the uterus expands, the mother's center of gravity shifts, which can cause back pain and discomfort.
9. Mood changes: Many women experience mood swings or feel more emotional during the third trimester.
10. Preparation for labor and delivery: In the final weeks of pregnancy, the mother's body begins to prepare for labor and delivery, with the cervix dilating and the baby moving into position for birth.
11. Hormonal changes: Hormonal changes during the third trimester can lead to increased levels of progesterone, which can cause relaxation of the ligaments and joints, preparing the body for delivery.
12. Braxton Hicks contractions: These are practice contractions that help the uterus prepare for labor. They can be uncomfortable, but they are usually not painful.

It is important for pregnant women to receive regular prenatal care during the third trimester to monitor fetal growth, manage any symptoms or complications, and prepare for labor and delivery.

Hormonal changes and their effects on the body

During the third trimester of pregnancy, hormonal changes continue to occur in the body to prepare for childbirth and motherhood.

One of the most significant hormones during this time is progesterone, which continues to increase to support the growth of the fetus and prepare the body for childbirth. However, high levels of progesterone can also cause some uncomfortable symptoms, such as constipation, heartburn, and difficulty sleeping.

Another important hormone during the third trimester is oxytocin, which helps stimulate contractions during labor and also plays a role in bonding with the baby after birth. In the weeks leading up to childbirth, the body produces increasing amounts of oxytocin, which can cause Braxton Hicks contractions or "false labor" that can be uncomfortable or even painful.

Additionally, estrogen and human chorionic gonadotropin (hCG) levels may decrease during the third trimester, which can lead to a range of symptoms, including fatigue, mood swings, and fluid retention.

Common symptoms and how to manage them

During the third trimester, the body experiences some of the most noticeable changes of pregnancy. Hormonal changes during this time cause the uterus to expand and the baby to grow rapidly. As a result, there are several common symptoms that pregnant women may experience during the third trimester, including:

1. Braxton Hicks contractions: These are often referred to as "practice contractions" and are a normal part of the third trimester. They may be uncomfortable but are not typically painful and do not lead to labor.
2. Shortness of breath: As the uterus expands and pushes against the diaphragm, it can be difficult to take deep breaths. This is normal but can be uncomfortable.
3. Back pain: As the baby grows, the extra weight can cause strain on the lower back, leading to discomfort.
4. Swelling: Many women experience swelling in their feet, ankles, and hands during the third trimester. This is due to the increased pressure on the blood vessels and can be exacerbated by hot weather or standing for long periods.
5. Fatigue: As the body prepares for labor and delivery, it can be exhausting to carry the extra weight of the baby.

To manage these symptoms during the third trimester, pregnant women can take several steps, including:

1. Staying hydrated: Drinking plenty of water can help reduce swelling and keep the body functioning properly.
2. Resting frequently: Taking breaks throughout the day to rest and elevate the feet can help reduce swelling and fatigue.

3. Practicing good posture: Maintaining good posture can help reduce back pain and prevent further strain on the body.
4. Doing prenatal yoga or other gentle exercise: Exercise can help maintain strength and flexibility and prepare the body for labor.
5. Talking to a healthcare provider: If symptoms are severe or concerning, pregnant women should talk to their healthcare provider for additional guidance and support.

Nutritional needs and dietary recommendations

During the third trimester, it is important to continue following a healthy and balanced diet to ensure the proper growth and development of the baby. The caloric needs of a pregnant woman increase during the third trimester, and it is recommended to consume an additional 300-500 calories per day.

Protein is especially important during the third trimester as it is necessary for the growth and development of the baby's tissues. Good sources of protein include lean meats, poultry, fish, eggs, legumes, nuts, and seeds.

Calcium and vitamin D are also important during the third trimester for the development of the baby's bones and teeth. Good sources of calcium include dairy products, dark leafy greens, fortified cereals, and calcium-fortified orange juice. Vitamin D is found in fatty fish, egg yolks, and fortified dairy products.

Iron is another important nutrient during the third trimester as it is needed to make hemoglobin, which carries oxygen to the baby. Good sources of iron include lean red meat, poultry, fish, iron-fortified cereals, and dark leafy greens. It is recommended to consume iron-rich foods with vitamin C-rich foods to enhance iron absorption.

It is also important to stay hydrated during the third trimester by drinking plenty of water and other fluids such as milk and 100% fruit juice.

It is important to discuss any dietary concerns or questions with a healthcare provider to ensure that all nutritional needs are being met during pregnancy.

Exercise and physical activity recommendations

During the third trimester, exercise and physical activity can become more challenging due to the growing size and weight of the baby, as well as the physical changes in the mother's body. However, it is still important to continue exercising for both the mother's and baby's health.

Here are some exercise and physical activity recommendations for the third trimester:

1. Walking: Walking is a low-impact exercise that can be done throughout the entire pregnancy. It helps to maintain cardiovascular health, improves circulation, and prepares the body for labor and delivery.

2. Prenatal yoga: Prenatal yoga can help to improve flexibility, balance, and circulation, while also reducing stress and promoting relaxation.
3. Swimming: Swimming is a low-impact exercise that can help to relieve pressure on the joints and back, while also providing a full-body workout.
4. Pelvic floor exercises: Pelvic floor exercises, also known as Kegels, help to strengthen the pelvic floor muscles, which can become weakened during pregnancy and childbirth.
5. Strength training: Strength training can help to maintain muscle tone and strength, which can be beneficial during labor and delivery.

It is important to listen to your body and avoid any exercises or physical activities that cause discomfort or pain. It is also recommended to consult with your healthcare provider before starting any new exercise routine during pregnancy.

Hormonal Imbalance during Pregnancy

During pregnancy, the body experiences a significant increase in hormonal activity, which can lead to hormonal imbalances. Hormones play a vital role in maintaining the pregnancy and supporting fetal development, but the hormonal changes that occur during pregnancy can also cause a range of physical and emotional symptoms.

Some of the hormones that are active during pregnancy include:

1. Human chorionic gonadotropin (HCG): This hormone is produced by the placenta and helps to maintain the pregnancy.
2. Progesterone: Progesterone helps to thicken the lining of the uterus, preparing it for implantation of the fertilized egg. It also helps to maintain the pregnancy by relaxing the muscles of the uterus.
3. Estrogen: Estrogen plays a role in fetal development and helps to prepare the breasts for lactation.
4. Relaxing: Relaxing is produced by the placenta and helps to relax the muscles and ligaments in the body in preparation for childbirth.
5. Prolactin: Prolactin is produced by the pituitary gland and helps to stimulate milk production after childbirth.

Hormonal imbalances during pregnancy can cause a range of symptoms, including:

1. Mood swings: Hormonal changes can cause mood swings, anxiety, and depression.
2. Fatigue: Increased levels of progesterone can cause fatigue, particularly in the first and third trimesters.
3. Nausea and vomiting: Hormonal changes can cause morning sickness, which is characterized by nausea and vomiting.
4. Constipation: Progesterone can slow down the digestive system, leading to constipation.
5. Insomnia: Hormonal changes can interfere with sleep, leading to insomnia.
6. Skin changes: Hormonal changes can cause acne, darkening of the skin, and skin tags.

7. Swelling: Increased levels of progesterone can cause fluid retention and swelling in the hands, feet, and ankles.

It is important to discuss any symptoms with a healthcare provider to ensure that they are not indicative of a more serious issue. In some cases, hormonal imbalances during pregnancy can lead to complications such as preterm labor, gestational diabetes, or preeclampsia.

Explanation of hormonal changes during pregnancy and their effects on the body

During pregnancy, the body undergoes a series of hormonal changes to support the development and growth of the fetus. These hormonal changes are necessary for a healthy pregnancy and delivery, but they can also lead to imbalances in the body, which can cause discomfort and health issues for the mother.

The main hormones involved in pregnancy are estrogen, progesterone, and human chorionic gonadotropin (hCG). In the early stages of pregnancy, the placenta produces small amounts of estrogen and progesterone, which increase significantly as the pregnancy progresses. These hormones are responsible for several changes in the body, including:

1. Growth and development of the fetus: Estrogen and progesterone stimulate the growth of the fetus and the development of the placenta, which provides nutrients and oxygen to the fetus.

2. Changes in the reproductive system: Estrogen and progesterone prepare the uterus for pregnancy by thickening the uterine lining and relaxing the muscles in the uterus.
3. Changes in other organs: Estrogen and progesterone also affect other organs, such as the breasts and the digestive system, during pregnancy.
4. Prevention of premature labor: Progesterone helps prevent premature labor by relaxing the muscles in the uterus.

HCG is another hormone that is produced during pregnancy. It is produced by the placenta and is responsible for maintaining the production of estrogen and progesterone. HCG levels increase rapidly in the first few weeks of pregnancy and are used to confirm pregnancy in pregnancy tests.

While these hormonal changes are necessary for a healthy pregnancy, they can also cause imbalances in the body, which can lead to several health issues for the mother. **Some common hormonal imbalances during pregnancy include:**

1. Morning sickness: Morning sickness is caused by increased levels of estrogen and hCG in the body. Symptoms include nausea, vomiting, and fatigue.
2. Mood swings: Hormonal changes during pregnancy can cause mood swings and emotional changes in some women.

3. Gestational diabetes: The hormonal changes during pregnancy can cause insulin resistance in some women, leading to gestational diabetes.
4. Pre-eclampsia: Pre-eclampsia is a condition that can occur in late pregnancy, characterized by high blood pressure and protein in the urine. It is thought to be caused by imbalances in hormones and blood vessels.
5. Thyroid problems: Pregnancy can cause imbalances in thyroid hormones, leading to hyperthyroidism or hypothyroidism.

It is important for pregnant women to have regular prenatal care to monitor these hormonal changes and ensure a healthy pregnancy.

Common hormonal imbalances during pregnancy and their symptoms

During pregnancy, hormonal imbalances can occur due to the significant changes that happen in the body. These hormonal imbalances can cause several symptoms that can affect a woman's overall well-being. Some of the most common hormonal imbalances during pregnancy include:

1. Estrogen and progesterone imbalances: Estrogen and progesterone are two crucial hormones during pregnancy. Imbalances in these hormones can lead to several symptoms, such as mood swings, fatigue, bloating, breast tenderness, and nausea.
2. Thyroid imbalances: The thyroid gland produces hormones that help regulate metabolism and energy levels. Hormonal

imbalances in the thyroid gland can cause several symptoms, including fatigue, weight gain, constipation, and dry skin.
3. Insulin imbalances: Insulin is a hormone that regulates blood sugar levels. During pregnancy, insulin resistance can occur, leading to high blood sugar levels and increasing the risk of gestational diabetes.
4. Cortisol imbalances: Cortisol is a hormone produced by the adrenal glands, which helps the body respond to stress. Hormonal imbalances in cortisol can cause several symptoms, including anxiety, depression, and high blood pressure.
5. Prolactin imbalances: Prolactin is a hormone that plays a crucial role in breast milk production. Hormonal imbalances in prolactin can cause several symptoms, including breast tenderness, decreased libido, and irregular menstrual periods.

It is important to note that some of these symptoms are common during pregnancy and may not always be due to hormonal imbalances. However, if you experience any unusual or severe symptoms, it is essential to consult your healthcare provider.

How to manage hormonal imbalances during pregnancy

Managing hormonal imbalances during pregnancy is important to ensure the health and well-being of both the mother and the baby. Here are some tips for managing hormonal imbalances during pregnancy:

1. Talk to your healthcare provider: If you are experiencing symptoms of hormonal imbalances, it is important to talk to your healthcare provider. They can help diagnose the issue and provide guidance on treatment options.
2. Eat a healthy diet: Eating a balanced and healthy diet is important during pregnancy, and can also help manage hormonal imbalances. Focus on consuming plenty of fruits, vegetables, lean proteins, and whole grains.
3. Stay hydrated: Drinking plenty of water can help regulate hormone levels and prevent dehydration, which can exacerbate hormonal imbalances.
4. Get enough sleep: Getting enough sleep is important for regulating hormone levels and managing stress, which can impact hormonal balance.
5. Manage stress: Stress can impact hormone levels, so it is important to practice stress-reducing techniques such as meditation, deep breathing, or yoga.
6. Consider natural remedies: Some natural remedies, such as essential oils or herbal supplements, may be effective in managing hormonal imbalances during pregnancy. However, it is important to talk to your healthcare provider before trying any new remedies.
7. Take medications as prescribed: If hormonal imbalances require medical treatment, it is important to take any prescribed medications as directed by your healthcare provider.

It is important to remember that hormonal imbalances during pregnancy are common and manageable. By taking care of yourself and working closely with your healthcare provider, you can manage hormonal imbalances and ensure a healthy pregnancy.

Complications during Pregnancy

Complications during pregnancy are unexpected health issues that arise during pregnancy, which can affect the health of the mother, the developing fetus, or both. While most pregnancies are healthy, some women may experience complications during pregnancy. Some common complications during pregnancy include:

1. Gestational Diabetes: Gestational diabetes is a type of diabetes that develops during pregnancy. It occurs when the body is unable to produce enough insulin to regulate blood sugar levels during pregnancy. Gestational diabetes can increase the risk of preterm labor, preeclampsia, and delivery complications.
2. Preterm Labor: Preterm labor is when contractions begin before 37 weeks of pregnancy. This can cause premature birth and may lead to complications for the baby, including respiratory distress, cerebral palsy, and developmental delays.
3. Preeclampsia: Preeclampsia is a condition that can occur after the 20th week of pregnancy. It is characterized by high blood pressure and protein in the urine. If left untreated, it can lead to serious complications for both the mother and baby, including seizures, stroke, and even death.
4. Miscarriage: A miscarriage is the loss of a pregnancy before the 20th week. Miscarriages can be caused by a variety of factors, including genetic abnormalities, hormonal imbalances, and health conditions in the mother.

5. Ectopic Pregnancy: An ectopic pregnancy occurs when the fertilized egg implants outside of the uterus, usually in the fallopian tube. Ectopic pregnancies can be life-threatening if not diagnosed and treated promptly.
6. Placenta Previa: Placenta previa is a condition in which the placenta partially or completely covers the cervix, which can cause bleeding during pregnancy and delivery.
7. Placental Abruption: Placental abruption is a serious condition in which the placenta separates from the uterine wall before delivery. This can cause heavy bleeding and can be life-threatening for both the mother and baby.
8. Group B Strep: Group B strep (GBS) is a bacterial infection that can be passed from mother to baby during delivery. It can cause serious infections in the baby, including sepsis and meningitis.
9. Birth Defects: Birth defects are abnormalities that occur in the baby's development before birth. They can be caused by genetic factors, environmental factors, or a combination of both.

It is important to note that not all complications can be prevented, but regular prenatal care can help identify and manage any issues that arise during pregnancy. If you experience any unusual symptoms or complications during pregnancy, it is important to seek medical attention right away.

Overview of common complications during pregnancy

During pregnancy, women may experience various complications that can affect their health as well as the health of the developing fetus. These complications can range from minor discomforts to serious conditions that require medical intervention. Some of the most common complications during pregnancy include:

1. Gestational diabetes: This is a type of diabetes that develops during pregnancy and can cause high blood sugar levels in the mother, which can affect the growth and development of the fetus.
2. Pre-eclampsia: This is a condition that causes high blood pressure and damage to organs, such as the liver and kidneys. If left untreated, it can lead to serious complications for both the mother and baby.
3. Miscarriage: This is the loss of a pregnancy before the 20th week. Miscarriages can occur due to various reasons such as chromosomal abnormalities, hormonal imbalances, and certain infections.
4. Ectopic pregnancy: This is a condition where the fertilized egg implants outside the uterus, usually in the fallopian tube. Ectopic pregnancies can be life-threatening and require immediate medical attention.
5. Placenta previa: This is a condition where the placenta is located low in the uterus and covers the cervix, which can cause bleeding and potentially harm the baby.
6. Preterm labor: This is when labor begins before the 37th week of pregnancy. Preterm labor can lead to premature birth, which can cause various complications for the baby.
7. Gestational hypertension: This is high blood pressure that develops during pregnancy and can cause complications for both the mother and baby.
8. Intrauterine growth restriction (IUGR): This is a condition where the fetus does not grow at a normal rate and can

lead to various complications for the baby, such as low birth weight and developmental delays.

9. Preeclampsia: This is a pregnancy complication characterized by high blood pressure and damage to organs, such as the liver and kidneys. It can cause serious complications for both the mother and baby, including seizures and premature delivery.

10. Placental abruption: This is a serious pregnancy complication where the placenta separates from the uterine wall before the baby is born, which can cause heavy bleeding and potentially harm the baby.

It's important for pregnant women to attend all prenatal appointments to detect and manage any potential complications as early as possible.

Signs and symptoms of complications

Signs and symptoms of complications during pregnancy can vary depending on the specific complication. However, some general signs and symptoms to look out for include:

1. Vaginal bleeding or spotting: This can be a sign of miscarriage, ectopic pregnancy, or placental problems.
2. Abdominal pain or cramping: This can be a sign of miscarriage, preterm labor, or placental problems.
3. Decreased fetal movement: This can be a sign of fetal distress.

4. Severe headache, blurred vision, or dizziness: These can be signs of preeclampsia, a serious condition that can lead to complications for both the mother and the baby.
5. Severe nausea and vomiting: This can be a sign of hyperemesis gravidarum, a condition that causes severe vomiting and can lead to dehydration and malnutrition.
6. High fever or chills: These can be signs of an infection, such as a urinary tract infection or pneumonia.
7. Swelling or puffiness in the face or hands: This can be a sign of preeclampsia or other complications.
8. Persistent contractions: This can be a sign of preterm labor.

If you experience any of these symptoms or are concerned about any changes in your body during pregnancy, it is important to contact your healthcare provider right away. Early intervention and treatment can often prevent or manage complications during pregnancy.

Treatment options for complications

The treatment options for complications during pregnancy depend on the type and severity of the complication. In some cases, no treatment may be needed, while in others, immediate medical attention may be required. Here are some common treatment options for complications during pregnancy:

1. Bed rest: For some complications, such as preterm labor or preeclampsia, bed rest may be recommended to help

manage symptoms and reduce the risk of further
complications.

2. Medications: Depending on the type of complication, medications may be prescribed to manage symptoms or treat the underlying condition. For example, antibiotics may be used to treat infections, while medications to lower blood pressure may be used to manage preeclampsia.

3. Surgery: In some cases, surgery may be necessary to treat complications during pregnancy. For example, if a woman experiences an ectopic pregnancy, surgery may be needed to remove the fetus and prevent further complications.

4. Lifestyle changes: Making lifestyle changes, such as quitting smoking or reducing stress, may be recommended to help manage or prevent complications during pregnancy.

5. Delivery: In some cases, delivering the baby may be the best course of action to prevent further complications. For example, if a woman experiences severe preeclampsia or placenta previa, delivery may be necessary to ensure the health and safety of both the mother and baby.

It is important to seek medical attention if you experience any symptoms of complications during pregnancy. Early detection and treatment can help prevent further complications and ensure the health and safety of both the mother and baby.

Prevention strategies for complications

There are several strategies that can help prevent complications during pregnancy, including:

1. Regular prenatal care: Attending regular prenatal appointments with a healthcare provider is important for monitoring the health of both the mother and baby and identifying any potential complications early.
2. Healthy lifestyle: Maintaining a healthy lifestyle by eating a balanced diet, staying physically active, getting enough rest, and avoiding harmful substances such as alcohol and tobacco can help reduce the risk of complications.
3. Managing chronic health conditions: Women with chronic health conditions such as diabetes, high blood pressure, or thyroid disorders should work closely with their healthcare provider to manage these conditions during pregnancy.
4. Genetic counseling: Women with a family history of genetic disorders or who are at increased risk for certain genetic conditions may benefit from genetic counseling to assess their risk and develop a plan for monitoring and managing any potential complications.
5. Understanding warning signs: Knowing the warning signs of potential complications, such as vaginal bleeding, severe abdominal pain, or decreased fetal movement, can help women seek prompt medical attention if necessary.

By taking steps to prevent complications and seeking timely medical care when necessary, women can help ensure a healthy pregnancy and delivery for themselves and their babies.

Tips for Staying Healthy During Pregnancy

Sure, here are some tips for staying healthy during pregnancy:

1. Eat a well-balanced diet: During pregnancy, it's important to consume a variety of nutrient-dense foods to support the growth and development of the baby. Aim to eat plenty of fruits, vegetables, whole grains, lean proteins, and healthy fats.
2. Stay hydrated: Drink plenty of water and avoid sugary drinks, which can add unnecessary calories and contribute to gestational diabetes.
3. Exercise regularly: Exercise can help you manage weight gain, reduce stress, and prepare your body for labor and delivery. Talk to your healthcare provider about what types of exercise are safe for you.
4. Get enough rest: It's important to get plenty of sleep during pregnancy, as your body is working hard to support the growth and development of your baby. Try to aim for 7-8 hours of sleep each night.
5. Manage stress: Stress can have negative effects on your pregnancy and your overall health. Try to incorporate relaxation techniques such as meditation, deep breathing, or yoga into your daily routine.
6. Attend prenatal appointments: Regular prenatal appointments are important to monitor the health and development of both you and your baby. Be sure to attend all appointments and communicate with your healthcare provider about any concerns you may have.
7. Avoid smoking, alcohol, and drugs: These substances can have negative effects on your baby's development and should be avoided during pregnancy.
8. Practice good hygiene: Wash your hands frequently to avoid getting sick, and avoid contact with anyone who is sick. Additionally, be sure to follow any guidelines provided

by your healthcare provider regarding COVID-19 precautions.

Remember, every pregnancy is different, so it's important to communicate with your healthcare provider about any concerns you may have and follow their recommendations for a healthy pregnancy.

Importance of regular prenatal care

Regular prenatal care is essential for ensuring a healthy pregnancy and a healthy baby. Prenatal care involves regular check-ups with a healthcare provider, such as an obstetrician or midwife, to monitor the health of both the mother and the developing fetus.

During prenatal care appointments, healthcare providers will monitor the mother's blood pressure, weight gain, and the baby's growth and development. They will also screen for any potential complications or health issues that may arise during pregnancy, such as gestational diabetes or preeclampsia.

Prenatal care also involves receiving important medical tests and procedures, such as ultrasounds, blood tests, and screenings for genetic disorders. These tests can help detect potential health issues early on, which can increase the chances of successful treatment and a healthy outcome for both mother and baby.

Overall, regular prenatal care is crucial for ensuring the best possible health outcomes for both mother and baby, and should be a top priority for all pregnant women.

Maintaining a healthy diet and exercise routine

Maintaining a healthy diet and exercise routine is crucial for a healthy pregnancy. Eating a balanced and nutritious diet and engaging in regular physical activity can help ensure the proper development of the fetus, reduce the risk of complications, and promote the overall health of the mother.

A healthy pregnancy diet should include a variety of nutrient-dense foods, including whole grains, fruits, vegetables, lean proteins, and healthy fats. It's also important to stay hydrated by drinking plenty of water and other fluids throughout the day. Avoiding processed and high-sugar foods is recommended.

Exercise during pregnancy is safe and beneficial for both the mother and the fetus. Regular physical activity can help reduce the risk of gestational diabetes, preeclampsia, and cesarean delivery. It can also help improve circulation, boost energy levels, and reduce stress and anxiety.

The American College of Obstetricians and Gynecologists (ACOG) recommends that pregnant women engage in at least 150 minutes of moderate-intensity aerobic exercise per week. Some examples of safe and effective exercises during pregnancy include brisk walking, swimming, prenatal yoga, and low-impact aerobics.

It's important to consult with a healthcare provider before beginning any exercise routine during pregnancy and to listen to your body's cues. Avoid exercises that cause discomfort or pain, and stop exercising immediately if you experience any bleeding, dizziness, or other concerning symptoms.

Managing stress and getting enough rest

Managing stress and getting enough rest are important for staying healthy during pregnancy. The physical and emotional stress of pregnancy can take a toll on the body, and chronic stress can increase the risk of complications like preterm labor, low birth weight, and preeclampsia. Getting enough rest and relaxation can help reduce stress and support the health of both the mother and baby.

Here are some tips for managing stress and getting enough rest during pregnancy:

1. Practice relaxation techniques: Relaxation techniques like deep breathing, meditation, and prenatal yoga can help reduce stress and promote relaxation.
2. Get enough sleep: Aim for 7-9 hours of sleep each night, and try to establish a consistent sleep routine. Avoid electronics and stimulating activities before bed.
3. Take breaks throughout the day: Take breaks throughout the day to rest and recharge. Try to incorporate relaxation

techniques into your breaks, like deep breathing or stretching.
4. Manage your workload: Avoid taking on too many responsibilities, and try to delegate tasks when possible.
5. Stay connected with loved ones: Having a support network of loved ones can help reduce stress and provide emotional support during pregnancy.
6. Seek professional help if needed: If you're struggling to manage stress on your own, consider seeking professional help from a therapist or counselor who specializes in prenatal mental health.

Avoiding harmful substances and environmental factors

During pregnancy, it is essential to avoid exposure to harmful substances and environmental factors that can adversely affect the health of the mother and the developing baby. Here are some tips for avoiding harmful substances and environmental factors:

1. Tobacco: Smoking during pregnancy can lead to premature birth, low birth weight, and a higher risk of sudden infant death syndrome (SIDS). If you are a smoker, quitting is the best thing you can do for your baby's health.
2. Alcohol: Drinking alcohol during pregnancy can cause fetal alcohol syndrome, which can result in lifelong physical and mental disabilities. It's best to avoid alcohol altogether during pregnancy.
3. Drugs: Using illegal drugs or abusing prescription drugs during pregnancy can cause a range of problems for the baby, including low birth weight, premature birth, birth

defects, and withdrawal symptoms. If you are struggling with addiction, seek help from your healthcare provider.

4. Environmental toxins: Exposure to certain chemicals and pollutants can be harmful to the developing fetus. To reduce your exposure, avoid using harsh cleaning products, pesticides, and other chemicals. Also, be cautious when eating certain types of fish that may contain high levels of mercury.

5. Radiation: High levels of radiation exposure can be harmful to the developing fetus. If you work in an industry that exposes you to radiation, talk to your healthcare provider about ways to reduce your exposure.

6. Heat: High temperatures can be harmful during pregnancy, particularly in the first trimester when the baby's neural tube is developing. Avoid spending time in saunas and hot tubs, and be careful not to overheat during exercise or in hot weather.

7. Stress: Chronic stress during pregnancy can increase the risk of preterm labor and low birth weight. Practice stress-reducing techniques like meditation, deep breathing, and gentle exercise to help manage stress during pregnancy.

Conclusion

In conclusion, pregnancy is a beautiful and exciting experience, but it can also be challenging for many women. It is important to prioritize your health and well-being throughout the three trimesters of pregnancy. By understanding the changes your body is undergoing and taking steps to manage symptoms and address hormonal imbalances, you can help ensure a healthy pregnancy and delivery.

Maintaining a healthy diet, getting regular exercise, managing stress, getting enough rest, and avoiding harmful substances are all key components of a healthy pregnancy. It is also important to seek regular prenatal care and to be aware of the signs and symptoms of potential complications.

Remember that every woman's pregnancy journey is unique, and it is important to listen to your body and seek guidance from your healthcare provider as needed. With the right care and attention, you can help ensure a healthy and happy pregnancy for both you and your baby.

Summary of key points

- Pregnancy is a period of significant physical and emotional changes in a woman's body.
- Staying healthy during pregnancy is essential for the well-being of both the mother and the baby.
- Pregnancy is divided into three trimesters, each with its unique characteristics and requirements.
- The first trimester is characterized by hormonal changes that can cause common symptoms like morning sickness, fatigue, and mood swings.
- The second trimester is often considered the easiest trimester because many women experience relief from the symptoms they experienced in the first trimester.

- The third trimester is characterized by more physical discomfort, including back pain, shortness of breath, and difficulty sleeping.
- Hormonal imbalances during pregnancy can cause various symptoms, including mood swings, fatigue, and changes in appetite.
- Common complications during pregnancy include gestational diabetes, preeclampsia, and preterm labor.
- Maintaining a healthy diet and exercise routine, managing stress, getting enough rest, avoiding harmful substances and environmental factors, and regular prenatal care are crucial for a healthy pregnancy.
- It is essential to seek medical attention promptly if any complications arise during pregnancy.

Overall, the key to a healthy pregnancy is to take care of yourself physically, emotionally, and mentally.

Importance of staying healthy during pregnancy for the mother and baby

Staying healthy during pregnancy is crucial for the well-being of both the mother and the baby. Eating a balanced diet, staying physically active, managing stress, getting enough rest, avoiding harmful substances and environmental factors, and seeking regular prenatal care are all essential for a healthy pregnancy.

The three trimesters of pregnancy each come with their own unique changes and challenges, including hormonal changes and associated symptoms. Hormonal imbalances can occur during pregnancy and may lead to additional symptoms such as mood swings, depression, and anxiety.

Complications during pregnancy can also arise, making it important to be aware of signs and symptoms and to seek medical attention when necessary. However, by following healthy habits and seeking regular prenatal care, many complications can be prevented or managed effectively.

Overall, the importance of staying healthy during pregnancy cannot be overstated. By taking care of oneself and following recommended guidelines, both mother and baby can experience a healthy pregnancy and a positive start to life.